YOUR KNOWLEDGE HAS VALUE

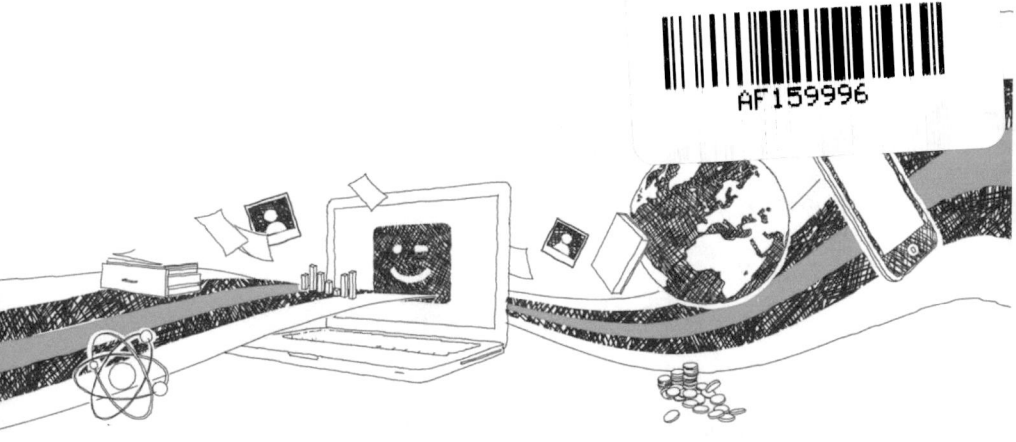

- We will publish your bachelor's and master's thesis, essays and papers

- Your own eBook and book - sold worldwide in all relevant shops

- Earn money with each sale

Upload your text at www.GRIN.com
and publish for free

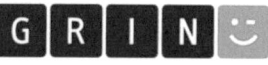

Bibliographic information published by the German National Library:

The German National Library lists this publication in the National Bibliography; detailed bibliographic data are available on the Internet at http://dnb.dnb.de .

This book is copyright material and must not be copied, reproduced, transferred, distributed, leased, licensed or publicly performed or used in any way except as specifically permitted in writing by the publishers, as allowed under the terms and conditions under which it was purchased or as strictly permitted by applicable copyright law. Any unauthorized distribution or use of this text may be a direct infringement of the author s and publisher s rights and those responsible may be liable in law accordingly.

Imprint:

Copyright © 2015 GRIN Verlag, Open Publishing GmbH
Print and binding: Books on Demand GmbH, Norderstedt Germany
ISBN: 9783668276178

This book at GRIN:

http://www.grin.com/en/e-book/337855/lower-back-pain-among-nurses-an-occupational-study-on-nurses-in-selected

Lok Raj Joshi, Sajana Shrestha

Lower back pain among nurses. An Occupational Study on Nurses in selected hospitals of Kathmandu, Nepal

GRIN Publishing

GRIN - Your knowledge has value

Since its foundation in 1998, GRIN has specialized in publishing academic texts by students, college teachers and other academics as e-book and printed book. The website www.grin.com is an ideal platform for presenting term papers, final papers, scientific essays, dissertations and specialist books.

Visit us on the internet:

http://www.grin.com/

http://www.facebook.com/grincom

http://www.twitter.com/grin_com

LOW BACK PAIN AMONG NURSES IN SELECTED HOSPITALS OF KATHMANDU, NEPAL

Nursing is considered as caring as well as challenging profession as nurses have to cope with many diverse situations from simple to complex work. This increasing competition and work demand put pressure on nurses physically and psychologically along with a high risk for occupational health problem. Low back pain (LBP) is commonest one. Thus, this study aimed to find out status & factors affecting LBP among nurses. Descriptive cross sectional study with verbal informed consent among 300 registered nurses by using simple random sampling was conducted. Semi structured questionnaires with Numeric Rating Scale (NRS) to measure severity of pain and Measure of Job Satisfaction (MJS), a likert scale to measure job satisfaction for psychological factors were used. Chi square test was used to see association. Among 300 nurses, prevalence of LBP was 68%. The mean age was 30.97±10.22 years. Among 240 nurses with LBP, severity was mild (37.3%). Long service duration >16 years (82.6%), prolong standing for 5-6 hours (73.1%), activity to provide nursing care (63.3%), not maintain good posture (58.1%) and prolong working hours of 47-52 hours/week (89.6%) were factors affecting LBP. MJS scale score was 2.96±0.878 which means subjects were neither satisfied nor dissatisfied. Significant association was found between long service duration, prolong working hours, incorrect posture, performing activity of nursing care and prolong standing. It is recommended to take appropriate measures to reduce long working hours, follow correct body mechanics, promote job satisfaction and to maintain standard nurse patient ratio to reduce work load to nurses in hospital settings.

Key words: Low back pain, Nurses, Body mechanics, Co-morbidities. Back trauma.

This text was written by a non-native English speaker. Please excuse any errors or inconsistencies.

CONTENT

INTRODUCTION 3
METHODS 3
RESULTS 4
    Table 1. Socio demographic characteristics 5
    Table 2. Pattern of low back pain (n=240) 6
    Table 3. Back pain arising posture (n=300) 7
    Table 4 Respondents' work pattern (n=300) 7
    Table 5. Association of factors with low back pain. (n=300) 8
DISCUSSION 8
CONCLUSION 10
AUTHOR STATEMENTS 11
REFERENCES 12

INTRODUCTION

Low back pain (LBP) is the most common and the leading category of occupational injury in health care or work-related health problem. Hospital workers experience more LBP than many other groups due to nature of their job.(1) Nurses play a major role in patient care. Nursing profession is one of the challenging professions as job demands in nursing is a mixture of physically (such as manual handling of patients) and mentally demanding tasks (such as dealing with crises).(2) A nurse has to provide 24 hours service in shift that implies either long term night work or work involving rotation between day, evening, and night shifts affecting disruption of circadian rhythm resulting in sleep disturbances, fatigue, and impaired work performance and safety awareness. They are always at risk for developing many occupational health problems like low back pain.(3) The etiology behind occupational LBP among nurses is usually multi factorial, which are physical factors (e.g. working in same position for longer periods, lifting or transferring dependent patient, heavy physical work, bending, twisting and caring for high number of patients.(4) and psychosocial factors (e.g. work environment, job content, job dissatisfaction, social support, personal relation). Therefore, occupational LBP is not only an individual medical problem, but also a global problem. (5)

Studies done among nurses worldwide showed the high prevalence of the condition reported at Bangladesh 66% in 2013,(6) Egypt 79.3% in 2012,(7) Taiwan 66% in 2007,(8). Annual prevalence reported at Switzerland 73%-76% in 2003, (9) Malaysia 56.9% in 2010(10). The consequences of LBP is responsible for poor quality of life, job absenteeism, high turnover decreased productivity of individual and national health services.(1) As Nepal is resource constraint country, low back pain is more prevalent in female health professional especially nurses that is affecting overall health services of Nepal likewise there is hardly any research regarding status of LBP among nurses in Nepal. Thus researcher aimed to conduct the research to find out the status of low back pain and factors affecting pain among the nurses of Nepal. Researcher expects that the findings of this research will help nursing professional to sensitize problem and early prevention of LBP in order to improve nations' health delivery services.

METHODS

Descriptive cross-sectional study was conducted in two hospitals, one government and another semi government hospital of Kathmandu from July to December 2014. Simple random sampling technique was used after making sampling frame of six government hospitals and three semi-governmental hospitals in Kathmandu based on document of list of hospitals published by Gelal Research Group on May 15, 2013. The study population was all nurses those who were registered nurse and registered Auxiliary nurse mid wife working in selected hospitals. Nurses who were physically and mentally unfit & have co-morbidities (arthritis, osteoporosis, ankylosing spondylitis, radicular syndrome or cauda equina syndrome, infection, inflammatory process, irritation, tumour & congenital abnormalities in the spine) or back trauma were excluded. Sample size was 345 which were determined by using the following formula.

$$n = \frac{z^2 pq}{d^2}$$

Where, n=sample size
Confidence limit (z) =1.96,
Nurses' prevalence with pain (p) =0.66, **[1]

---

[1] ** Prevalence (66%) was taken from a cross-sectional study among 100 nurses from three selected hospitals in Savar, Bangladesh in 2013 (6)

Acceptable Standard error (d) =0.05 (5%) &
Person's proportion of free of condition (q) = 1-p = 1- 0.66= 0.34.
Self-administered semi-structured questionnaire was used for data collection. Among 345 respondents, 300 (86.9%) responded so sample size was 300. Questions were translated into Nepali. All ethical issue was addressed according to ethical guidelines of State University of Bangladesh and concerned authority of organization. Administrative approval was taken from an organization. Verbal informed consent was taken from the respondent. Anonymity and confidentiality were maintained.

Questionnaire consists of four section related to socio demographic characteristics, pattern of pain (experience, timing, severity, distribution, duration, intensity of pain), factors of pain (physical, social, psychological and organizational factors) and work pattern of nurses. The factors that contribute to LBP i.e. socio demographic characteristics (age, BMI, marital status, service duration), physical factors (Incorrect posture, prolong standing), social factors (low job satisfaction, low support from seniors, relationship with co-workers), organizational factors (duty hours, night shift rate), work pattern (type of nursing activities, administrative working time) were taken as independent variable where as low back pain as dependent variable.

LBP is defined as symptom of a pain which can be localized at the precise anatomical delineation of spinal area of low back (between coastal margins of twelfth rib and the inferior gluteal folds), with or without radiating leg pain from various causes but is not a disease. Correct body mechanics is defined as keeping straight back, lifting chin, heading up while sitting and standing, bending knees while lifting low objects, avoiding twisting, keeping wide leg base support while standing.

Instrumentations were used to identify severity of pain measured by using the valid pain measurement scale called Numeric Rating Scale (NRS). It is a single segmented 11-point numeric scale in a horizontal bar or line that measures pain severity in adults where 0 representing one pain extreme (e.g., "no pain") and 10 representing the other pain extreme (e.g., "pain as bad as you can imagine" and "worst pain imaginable"). Job satisfaction level was measured by using valid and reliable tool named Measure of Job Satisfaction (MJS). It comprises 7 subscales; Personal satisfaction, Satisfaction with workload, Satisfaction with professional support, Satisfaction with training, Satisfaction with pay, Satisfaction with prospects, Satisfaction with standards of care which may be combined to give a measure of 'Overall Job Satisfaction'. There are 43 items and respondents were asked to rate their degree of job satisfaction on a five-point likert scale, ranging from 'very satisfied' to 'very dissatisfied'. Data analysis was done by using Statistical Package for Social Sciences (SPSS) version 16.0 & mean, frequency distribution, percentage etc. were used for analysis. Interpretation was done in frequency tables, pie charts & bar diagrams. Chi square test was applied to explain the association of age, service duration, working department, job satisfaction with low back pain.

RESULTS
Among 300 nurses who responded those of sample size 345 the prevalence was 68%. . Out of 300, more than half 156 (52%) were unmarried, 116 (38.7%) were Diploma in Nursing, only 8 (2.7%) were having M.Sc. or Master in Nursing. Nearly three fourth 217 (72.3%) were staff

nurse, 68 (22.7%) were Auxiliary Nurse Midwife and only 15 (5%) were Nurse In charge. (Table 1).

Table 1. Socio demographic characteristics

	F (%)
Marital Status	
Unmarried	156 (52%)
Married	108 (36%)
Widow	24 (8%)
Divorced	12 (4%)
Education	
Auxiliary Nurse Midwife course	68 (22.7%)
Diploma in Nursing	116 (38.6%)
B.Sc. or Post Basic Bachelor in Nsg	108 (36%)
M.Sc. or Master in Nursing	8 (2.7%)
Designation	
Auxiliary Nurse Midwife	68 (22.7%)
Staff nurse	217 (72.3%)
Nurse In-charge	15 (5%)

Nearly one tenth (9.3%) were from cardiac ICU unit, 24 (8%) were from cardiac surgical and Female medical ward, 20 (6.7%) each were from ICU, Male medical ward I and II, Neurology, Male surgical and Female surgical wards. Orthopedic ward, Oncology ward Urology ward, Coronary Care Unit (CCU), Cardiac Medical ward and Cardiac emergency ward had 16 (5.3%) respondents each. Few 8 (2.7%) were from ENT ward.

Researcher tried to explore the severity of low back pain using Numeric Rating Scale (NRS). Among 300 respondents, severity of pain was mild in 112 (37.3%), 76 (25.3%) had pain moderate pain, 16 (5.3%) & 96 (32.1%) had severe pain & no pain respectively.

Table 2. Pattern of low back pain (n=240)

	F (%)
Distribution of pain	
Localized to lower back	148 (72.5%)
Radiated to buttock	32 (15.7%)
Radiated to leg	24 (11.8%)
Timing of pain	
During activity	96 (47.1%)
After activity	76 (37.2%)
All the times	32 (15.7%)
Duration of pain	
Less than 6 weeks	132 (64.7%)
6-12 weeks	28 (13.7%)
More than 12 weeks	44 (21.6%)
Intensity of pain	
No analgesics only rest	140 (68.6%)
Analgesics required	16 (7.8%)
Both analgesics & rest	32 (15.7%)
Not relieved by analgesics	16 (7.8%)
Pain occurring Shift	
Morning shift	132 (64.7%)
Evening shift	12 (5.9%)
Night shift	60 (29.4%)

Among pain positive respondents, pattern of low back pain showed nearly three fourth 148 (72.5%) had localized pain, 32 (15.7%) had pain radiated to buttock & 24 (11.8%) had pain radiated to leg. Most respondents 96 (47.1%) felt pain during activity, 76 (37.2%) felt after activity & 32 (15.7%) felt all the times. Nearly two third 132 (64.7%) were suffering from pain less than 6 weeks whereas 28 (13.7%) had pain between 6-12 weeks and 44 (21.6%) had pain more than 12 weeks. 140 (68.6%) had intensified pain that doesn't required analgesics only rest is sufficient, 32 (15.7%) required both analgesics and rest. Both requiring analgesics and whom pain is not even relieved by analgesics were same i.e 16 (7.8%). Almost two third, respondents 132 (64.7%) answered pain intensified most in morning shift, 60 (29.4%) in night shift and 12 (5.9%) in evening shift (Table 2).

Posture that aroused back pain was multiple responses. Nearly two third of the respondents 124 (63.3%) answered while performing nursing care procedure. 104 (53.1%) replied prolong standing, 80 (40.8%) answered bending, 40 (20.4%) while lifting patients and equipment & only 16 (8.2%) while pulling and pushing objects. (Table 3)

Table 3. Back pain arising posture (n=300)

Posture	**Response (%)
Prolong standing	104 (53.1%)
Prolong sitting	24 (12.2%)
Bending	80 (40.8%)
Lifting patient and equipment	40 (20.4%)
Pulling and pushing objects	16 (8.2)%
Providing nursing care procedures	124 (63.3%)
**Multiple responses	

Table 4 Respondents' work pattern (n=300)

Type of nursing activities	F (%)
Basic care	98 (32.7%)
Complex care	87 (29%)
Administrative work	35 (11.7%)
Clerical work	27 (9%)
Housekeeping work	22 (7.3%)
Maintaining supplies/equipments	31 (10.3%)
Administrative working time	
1-2 hours	199 (66.3%)
3-4 hours	93 (31%)
5-6 hours	8 (2.7%)

The results regarding work pattern of respondents includes type of nursing activity that is done in a shift duty. Among 300 respondents, nearly one third 98 (32.7%) did basic care, 87 (29%) did complex care and least 22 (7.3%) did housekeeping work.

Result time spent for administrative working depicted two third 199 (66.3%) of respondents spent 1-2 hours of administrative work whereas 93 (31.0%) spent 3-4 hours of administrative work. Minor 8 (2.7%) respondents spent 5-6 hours for administrative work. (Table 4)

Association of factors of pain with low back pain was done which were socio demographic factors (age, BMI & service duration), physical factors (frequency of maintenance of good posture, duration of standing), organizational factor (duty hours per week) & psychological factor (job satisfaction). Result showed there was statistically significant association ($p<0.05$) of factors of back pain (service duration, duty hours per week, maintenance of good posture, standing duration per shift and overall job satisfaction) with presence of low back pain. Likewise, results showed there is no statistically significant association ($P>0.05$) of age and BMI with the presence of low back pain. As the age and BMI of the respondent increases there is presence of respondents' back pain. (Table 5)

Table 5. Association of factors with low back pain. (n=300)

	LBP yes (N=204)	No LBP (N=96)	p-value
Age group			0.157
<20 years	20 (71.4%)	8 (28.6%)	
21-30 years	96 (61.5%)	60 (38.5%)	
31-40 years	48 (75%)	16 (25%)	
41-50 years	24 (75%)	8 (25%)	
>50 years	16 (80%)	4 (20%)	
BMI			0.619
Underweight	12 (60%)	8 (40%)	
Normal	156 (67.8%)	74 (32.2%)	
Overweight	36 (72%)	14 (28%)	
Service duration			0.001
<5 years	92 (57.5%)	68 (42.5%)	
5-10 years	46 (79.3%)	12 (20.7%)	
11-16 years	28 (77.8%)	8 (22.2%)	
> 16 years	38 (82.6%)	8 (17.4%)	
Duty hours/week			0.000
40-46 hours	10 (13%)	67 (87%)	
47-52 hours	155 (89.6%)	18 (10.4%)	
53-58 hours	39 (78%)	11 (22%)	
Maintain good posture			0.000
Always	20 (40.8%)	29 (59.2%)	
Frequently	91 (78.4%)	25 (21.6%)	
Occasionally	68 (73.9%)	24 (26.1%)	
Never	25 (58.1%)	18 (41.9%)	
Standing duration/shift			0.001
1-2 hours	64 (54.7%)	53 (45.3%)	
3-4 hours	91 (78.4%)	25 (21.6%)	
5-6 hours	49 (73.1%)	18 (26.9%)	
Overall job satisfaction			0.001
Very dissatisfied	4 (100%)	0 (0%)	
Dissatisfied	81 (76.4%)	25 (23.6%)	
Neither satisfied nor dissatisfied	66 (73.3%)	24 (26.7%)	
Satisfied	50 (51.5%)	47 (48.5%)	
Very satisfied	3 (100%)	0 (0%)	

DISCUSSION

LBP is a common cause of morbidity in health care workers. Nurses are among the occupational groups within the health service that are more vulnerable to LBP. Mechanical hazards in the hospitals include LBP from manual lifting (patients in particular) as well female oriented profession which makes nursing one of the occupations most affected by LBP. (11)

Current descriptive cross sectional study was designed to find out the status of low back pain among nurses in selected hospitals of Kathmandu. Pattern of low back pain, work and factor affecting low back pain was also explored. Sample size was 345 but only 300 registered nurses responded during study including Auxiliary Nurse Midwives, staff nurses and Nurse In charge those who were randomly selected as subjects in this study.

Present study shows prevalence of back pain was found to be 68% which is similar among nurses in Bangladesh which was 66% (6) and also in Taiwan (8) whereas much higher (79.3%) in Egypt (7). This might be because comparing countries are also developing countries like Nepal with limited resource, advanced technology and devices for patient's care. In this study, LBP was found four fifth (80%) among respondents more than 50 years of age. There was no significant association (p=0.157) between age and pain. The BMI (kg/m^2) results shows about three fourth (67.8%) were in normal range (<18.5 to ≥25) and there was no significant association (p=0.001). Different result was found in a study by El-Soud AMA. in Egypt in 2014 that revealed (48%) with normal range, 52% obese. (7) This might be because obesity is less problematic in Nepal than other African and European countries. Those working more than 16 years, (82.6%) had pain statistically high significant association (p<0.05) was found between service duration and pain. Corresponding findings on study by El-Soud AMA. in Egypt where those working 20 years or more, (86.1 %) had pain. Working duration was significantly associated with the most recent episode of back pain. (7)

Measuring severity was one of factor to detect pattern of pain by using Numeric Rating Scale which revealed mild pain as more prevalent i.e. nearly two fifth (37.3%) & only few (5.3%) had severe pain. A study in 2013 in Bangladesh by Rashid HA detected 30% mild pain which is similar to our study but almost double (13%) had severe pain. (6) This might be because most of subjects almost two third (64.7%) were at initial stage of pain having pain duration less than 6 weeks. Nearly half (47.1%) had experienced pain during activity.

The main physical factor affecting low back pain were following incorrect body posture (58.1%) while working, standing and sitting, prolong standing & performing nursing care procedure (53.1) and bending (40.8%). Similar study done in Nepal by Adhikari S. in 2014 also revealed prolong standing (87%), frequent bending and twisting (51%), lifting heavy load/patients (46%), awkward posture (36%) as topmost factors that increase LBP. (13). In our study, prolonged standing (p=0.001) & maintenance of good posture (p=0.000) was highly significant with LBP.

Performing more duty hours work (47-52 hours/week) was one of the major organizational factor affecting LBP resulting (10.4%) of respondents with pain. There was statistically high significant association (p=0.000) between duty hours/week and LBP. Similar findings was found in a study in Sudan in 2015 where working hours was significantly associated (P-0.015) with LBP (14) and also significantly associated in study by Yassi A in Canada in 2013 (15). In this study, those with pain, respondents' who need to do night shift (2 nights/week) was found in four fifth (84%) of respondents whereas 5% in 4 nights/week. Unalike outcome is found in study by Jane KJ. in 2010 where above three fourth (76%) did 6 nights/week and (24%) less than 6 nights/week. Working 6 or more night shifts per month were related to a 64% increase

(OR = 1·64; 95% CI = 1·16–2·33) and 48% increase (OR = 1·48; 95% CI = 1·10–1·99) in back pain, respectively. (16) Different result might be because subjects in comparing study were from ICU and this study was from both general and specific wards where there is less night shift with max. 4 nights per shift in organizational policy.

The one of the main psychological factor of LBP was job satisfaction which was measured by instrument named Measure of Job Satisfaction (MJS) scale. Results showed dissatisfaction of respondents towards working hours (37%), Leave, training service provision (54%), Patient care quality (36%) on the other hand two-fifth had satisfaction toward support and relationship with senior, co-worker & colleague. Among dissatisfied three fourth (76.4%) had pain which is statically high significant (p=0.001). Related findings was in study where low job security was significantly associated with LBP (OR 0.82; 95% CI, 0.69, 0.98) along with low job satisfaction (OR 0.71; 95% CI, 0.51, 0.97) and high job support (OR 1.35; 95% CI, 1.04, 1.75). Low job security was found independently associated with LBP, whereas negative beliefs, reduced job satisfaction, and high job support were independently related to time off work. (17). Similarity of result was in study a by Brahrami N in 2011 where satisfaction for patient care was high (31.5%) and relation with supervisor was low (16.25%) among pain respondents. (18) This study shows there is good relation among   supervisor, co-worker & colleague. Overall average satisfaction rate mean score was (2.96±0.878) which means respondents were neither satisfied nor dissatisfied. A study in 1993 which also uses measure of job satisfaction (MJS) scale revealed overall mean scores was 3.31±0.49 which means respondents were satisfied. (19)

The type nursing activity of work pattern depicted work performance of basic care by one-third (32.7%), (29%) with complex care, (11.7%) administrative work, (9%) clerical work and (10.3%) of the activity of maintaining of supplies and equipment and only (7.3%) did housekeeping work during duty shifts. Nearly two third (66.3%) of respondent spent 3-4 hour's time in administrative work. A study by Tamilselvi A. in India in 2013 revealed results of work activity as (6.2%) basic nursing care, (66.8%) complex nursing care, (4.1%) administration, (9.9%) clerical, (1.7%) housekeeping, (2.4%) maintenance and (8.7%) non-productive activity.(20) More than half of the nursing activities performed by staff nurses were complex nursing activities but in our study it was nearly half times low i.e. (29%). The reason for high respondents doing complex care might be because comparative study is done in medical ward and this study is in both general and critical ward.

CONCLUSION

Low back pain is the most common costly and the leading category of occupational problem in health care professional especially nursing profession in the developing countries like Nepal where there is lack of sophisticated resources in providing patient care.

Prevalence was found high. Pattern of low back pain was found with mild severity that occurs while doing activity, less intensified pain which requires rest with no analgesics occurring especially in morning shift. In major physical factors of pain, prevalence was found high among those not maintaining good posture, prolong standing, bending, lifting, providing patients care Working more hours was major organizational factors of LBP. Less job satisfaction level was major psychological factors of low back pain. LBP was more prevalent among those having more service duration. No significant association between age and pain & BMI and pain was found.

It is recommended that nurses should follow correct body mechanic while doing patient care. Measures to be taken by organization to reduce long working hours, promote job satisfaction level and to maintain standard nurse patient ratio to reduce work load to nurses.

AUTHOR STATEMENTS

This research was done with self-funding, no any person and organization directly or indirectly took part in the research funding. All ethical issue was addressed according to ethical guidelines of State University of Bangladesh and concerned authority of organization. Administrative approval was taken from an organization. Verbal informed consent was taken from the respondent. I will express my thanks to all the respondent as well the selected hospital for the better cooperation during this research.

REFERENCES
1. Lin PH, Tsai YA, Chen WC, Huang SF. Prevalence, characteristics, and work-related risk factors of low back pain among hospital nurses in Taiwan: a cross-sectional survey. Int J Occup Med Environ Health. 2012;25(1):41-50.

2. Westgaard RH. Effects of physical and mental stressors on muscle pain. Scandinavian Journal of Work, Environment & Health. 1999:19-24.

3. Trinkoff AM, Storr CL, Lipscomb JA. Physically demanding work and inadequate sleep, pain medication use, and absenteeism in registered nurses. Journal of Occupational and Environmental Medicine. 2001;43(4):355-63.

4. Tinubu BM, Mbada CE, Oyeyemi AL, Fabunmi AA. Work-related musculoskeletal disorders among nurses in Ibadan, South-west Nigeria: a cross-sectional survey. BMC Musculoskeletal disorders. 2010;11(1):1.

5. Guide to care for patients. Low back pain. Nurse Pract. 2009;34(5):19-20.

6. Harun-Ar-Rashid H. Prevalence of low back pain among the nurses: Department of Physiotherapy, Bangladesh Health Professions Institute, CRP; 2013.

7. El-Soud AMA, El-Najjar AR, El-Fattah NA, Hassan AA. Prevalence of low back pain in working nurses in Zagazig University Hospitals: an epidemiological study. Egyptian Rheumatology and Rehabilitation. 2014;41(3):109.

8. Feng CK, Chen ML, Mao IF. Prevalence of and risk factors for different measures of low back pain among female nursing aides in Taiwanese nursing homes. BMC Musculoskelet Disord. 2007;8:52.

9. Maul I, Läubli T, Klipstein A, Krueger H. Course of low back pain among nurses: a longitudinal study across eight years. Occupational and environmental medicine. 2003;60(7):497-503.

10. Wong T, Teo N, Kyaw M. Prevalence and risk factors associated with low back pain among health care providers in a district hospital. Malaysian Orthopaedic Journal. 2010;4(2):23-8.

11. Sikiru L, Hanifa S. Prevalence and risk factors of low back pain among nurses in a typical Nigerian hospital. 2010.

12. Tobaco control laws. WHO. feb5, 2007.

13. Adhikari S, Dhakal G. Prevalent Causes of Low Back Pain and its Impact among Nurses Working in Sahid Gangalal National Heart Centre. J Nepal Health Res Counc. 2014;12(28):167-71.

14. Al-samawi MAG, Awad HMAA. Prevelenace of low back pain among nurses working in elmak nimer university hospital–shendi-sudan. September 2015;3(9):108-21.

15. Yassi A, Lockhart K. Work relatedness of low back pain in nursing personnel: a systematic review. International journal of occupational and environmental health. 2013;19(3):223-44.

16. June KJ, Cho SH. Low back pain and work-related factors among nurses in intensive care units. J Clin Nurs. 2011;20(3-4):479-87.

17. Urquhart DM, Kelsall HL, Hoe VCW, Cicuttini FM, Forbes AB, Sim MR. Are Psychosocial Factors Associated With Low Back Pain and Work Absence for Low Back Pain in an Occupational Cohort? The Clinical Journal of Pain. 2013;29(12):1015-20.

18. Bahrami N, Hojjati H, Hosseine FH. Relationship between backache and psychological and psychosocial job factors among the nurses. International Journal of nursing and Midwifery. 2011;3(7):86-91.

19. Traynor M, Wade B. The development of a measure of job satisfaction for use in monitoring the morale of community nurses in four trusts. Journal of Advanced Nursing. 1993;18(1):127-36.

20. Tamilselvi A, Regunath R. Work sampling: A quantitative analysis of nursing activity in a medical ward. Nitte University Journal of Health Science. 2013;3(3).

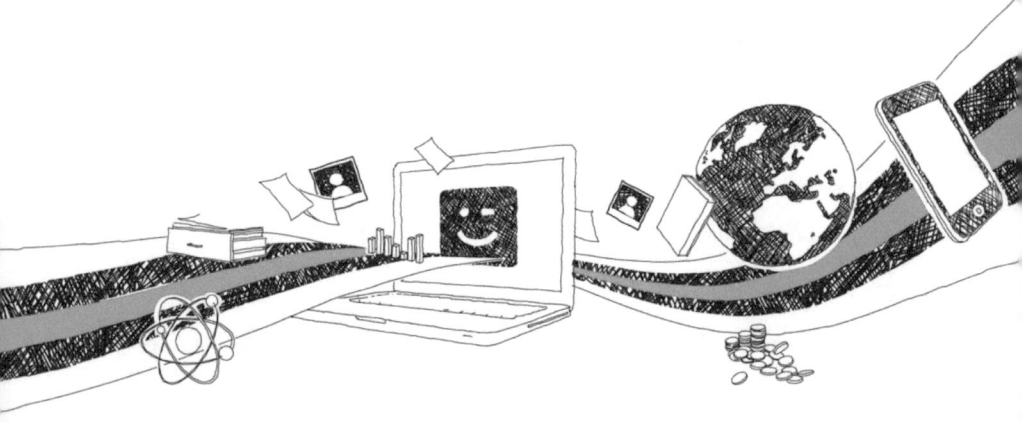